JUST MOM

A journey of love and laughter

Just Mom

Just Mom—A Journey of Love and Laughter
©2019 by Beverly Carriere Tiner

All rights reserved. With the exception of brief excerpts for review purposes, no portion of this book or its cover art may be reproduced or used in any form without written permission from the author.

All scripture quotations are taken from the NLT of the Bible.

Cover design: Beverly Carriere Tiner

Printed in The United States of America
First Edition 2019

ISBN: 9781094693071
Independently published

Beverly Carriere Tiner

For Mark,
the one whom my soul loves.
Thank you for holding my hand, and hers.

Just Mom

Beverly Carriere Tiner

THE FIRST YEAR

Just Mom

My mother's 6-week stint in the rehabilitation facility, after her mysterious collapse at home, was fast coming to a close. She had been diagnosed as "self-limiting". They had done all they could for her. To the therapists, that meant that when she wasn't "over-thinking", she was able to accomplish the objectives that they set before her. Other times, she seemingly wouldn't comply. She would lapse into confusion or delusions. As I sat with her throughout the days, she would tell me stories of things that happened in the night, things that, when I inquired of the rehab staff, they had no explanations for. She would occasionally awake, terrified, causing the staff to rely on medication to calm her down. In actuality, there was a disconnect manifesting in her brain that prevented her from functioning in a consistent manner. There was a monster causing her to see things that weren't there, to hear sounds that came from her own imagination. There was an intermittent glitch that caused her to forget the ones whom she knew best, then hours-or perhaps days later, remember them. There was a black hole that was actively sucking her very spirit into its abyss, leaving times of "black out" where she lost hours or sometimes, days. There was a run-away train that had taken her captive, a ride that she could not get off. That journey later became known as Lewy-Body Dementia.

I truly had no idea what I was in for. I remember speaking with one of the CNA's at the rehab who had been so kind to my mom, asking him if he thought I should, as had been suggested, put her into full-time nursing care, or follow my heart and bring her home. He looked at me with such compassion and said, "You can do this. *It's just Mom.*". I never forgot those words. It was my "love conquers all" moment. Against the advice of the doctors and many well-meaning friends and family, I brought my mother home to live with my husband and me and began my jaunt as a full-time caregiver. Together, we embarked on a journey that none of us had a clue about. We only knew that we loved each other and we would go through it together. Mom had been given about six months to live. I was determined to make them the best six months of her life.

What started as a six-month prognosis, turned into nearly 3-years. One of my own physicians, about a year into the journey, looked at me with concern and said, "you're giving away your years". Indeed, I was, years that I will cherish to my last breath, years that were filled with tears, but also laughter as we learned to navigate the unpredictable path of Lewy-Body. Those years were my gift to her, and, ultimately, hers to me. We adjusted accordingly, letting love be our guide. One thing I learned was that Lewy could take the mind and confound the body, but never ever could it take the love.

My mother was a realist. On her good days, we would have deep talks about her illness. She wanted to know what was happening to her. We had the same conversation many times. I promised never to lie to her. It helped her to feel safe, knowing that when she couldn't trust whatever she was seeing, hearing, or feeling, she could trust me. She could trust my husband. She knew we would protect her and care for her no matter what.

I found ways to ground her to reality. There was (and still is) a wall-paper border in her bedroom that she had actually helped to hang many years prior when that room belonged to one of my daughters. No matter what her delusion, she would always see that wallpaper border. It seemed to follow her on every "trip". One day, as we were discussing this, I told her to try to keep in her mind that, as long as she could see the green lattice border, she could be sure that she was safe in her bedroom, regardless of the delusion that her mind was conjuring. That green lattice border became her anchor until each crazy ride would pass. She also learned to ask me, "Is this real or am I imagining it?". It was a way for her to hang on to reality, to feel safe, until Lewy let go of her mind and allowed her to return to earth. She knew that if she could see the green lattice border or ask me that question, that she was safe. She was not alone, never alone.

She attached her off-beat, often dark humor to most days. I came to see her sense of humor as the gift that it was. Jesus gave us the strength to persevere, but laughter was like a burst of white energy that propelled us onward. I began to write down many of her daily quips. They now reside within the pages of this book. This book is a narrative of what was and what is; a journal of love and laughter--the best medicine for the worst times.

We brought Mom home to live with us in July of 2015. It wasn't long before she started referring to our home as "Bev's Care Center". She would comment on how peaceful it was, the "good care" she received, and the delicious food. The first few months were quite difficult as we tried to figure out what in the world was happening. As I learned that certain medications triggered her delusions, we began to take the most organic, holistic approach possible for her. She was weaned off most medication, any and all that would exacerbate her condition. Her diet was balanced and healthy. Her surroundings were peaceful. Her days were scheduled and predictable. It wasn't long before she was stabilized, with just the occasional delusion happening monthly, usually during the full-moon. Her doctor commented that she was healthier than he'd ever seen her.

Through it all, her sense of humor never wavered.

- ❖ Getting Mom ready for bed. She hands me her slippers. She hands me her glasses. Then, she says with a chuckle, "I'm gonna keep my teeth." *(Mom doesn't have dentures.).*

Just Mom

- ❖ As I'm cleaning up dinner, Mom shuffles by with her walker and says, "I'd help you with dishes, but I did them last night."

- ❖ As I was massaging one of my herbal healing oils into Mom's sore back, I said, "Maybe tomorrow will be better", to which she replied with great gusto, "there's no MAYBE about it! It's GOING to BE!"

- ❖ We were talking about birthdays, and Mom says, "I guess we've got all of our July birthdays done." I said, "Yeah, I think so." Then she said, "Wait, there are a lot more....but they're all dead!"

- ❖ Tonight, I asked Mom what she would do if she could do anything she wanted. She thought for a moment and said, "I don't know, probably help other people. That's what we're put here on earth for - to help each other."

- ❖ Mom is all situated in her chair watching the Price Is Right game show. Her back is sore. As I hand her a Tylenol, she says, "is that my prize?"

- ❖ All fed, dressed, and settled in her chair, I jokingly say to Mom, "now behave yourself." Her response? "Tomorrow."

- Mom takes one look at my chevron-printed skirt and says: "Boy! Your skirt makes me dizzy!".

- As I'm explaining to my mom that she needs to sit back in her recliner/lift chair before she pushes the recline control so that it recognizes that she's there (ie: a slow recline vs a sudden shift backward), she takes the controller in her hand and talks into it, "do you know I'm here??"

- Because my husband is our amazing, Mr. Fix-it, Jack-of-all-trades, and currently fixing his mom's well-pump, my mom sighs and says, "call Mark and see if he can fix ME!".

- I mentioned to Mom that she was talking in her sleep during her nap this afternoon, having a dream, but I don't know about what, she calmly responds, "well you should listen".

- I just turned to Mom and said, "Are you gonna clean up the kitchen tonight or am I?" She responded with, "I'll help you, but you won't find nothin".

- Mom, pushing her walker on the way to her room, slows down and gently eases it over the little threshold at her doorway and says, "speedbump!".

Just Mom

- ❖ Bella, my dog, has been sticking to me like glue...not sure if it's the stormy weather or she's just being my sweet, sensitive girl, but I mentioned it to mom and her response was, "maybe it's your pants (which were printed with a tropical, palm tree theme). She probably wants to pee on those trees."

- ❖ Our after-lunch conversation goes a little bit like this: Me: "I'm going to go wash dishes--or did you want to?" Mom: "I'm on vacation. (pause) I'll have an Almond Joy." Me: "Well, we don't have any Almond Joys." Mom: "Well, I want one." *She happily settled for a Hershey's Special Dark with Almonds.*

- ❖ I got mom all tucked into bed with a hug and a kiss and as I go to the door, I say, "I love you". She looks at me and says, "I love you, too" and shoots me a peace sign. *(2x the love).*

- ❖ Mom throws a tissue toward the trash can and misses, then says, "well, I won't have to hear about that--because I can't hear!" then laughs and laughs.

- ❖ As I'm helping Mom into bed, I hand her a tissue and mention that her eye is running. She takes it, dabs her eye and says, "I told you I cry every time you leave." *(followed by much laughter).*

❖ Mom has been having trouble blurring the line between me and my sister, Jean, who lives in another state. We were talking about it tonight as I was helping her get ready for bed. She had just called me "Jean" for the millionth time. I usually just look at her till she realizes the mistake or ignore it altogether. This time she realized it and said, "I don't know why I keep doing it, maybe because you have similar mannerisms; you're both funny." I said, "Well, I figure you named me, so you're allowed to call me whatever you want!" She laughed. After I gave her a kiss goodnight, I told her to call me if she needed anything. I closed the door and immediately hear a singsong voice say, "Bev-er-ly...". I open the door and she says, "Oh good! It works!" then busts out laughing!!!

❖ I was walking by the living room where Mom was sitting watching TV when I heard her say, "oh, SHUT UP!" I backed up and asked her who she was talking to. She pointed at the TV and said, "HIM!". It was a KIA commercial with the HUGE guy.

Everyone needs to be needed. We all need a sense of purpose. That need never goes away, even when someone is plagued by dementia. My mom was always doing for others. It was incredibly difficult for her to learn to be on the receiving end without feeling like a burden. She always felt like she needed to earn her keep. I reminded her almost daily that a burden is something that we don't want to carry. She was never that to me. The years of being her caregiver changed me, grew me, blessed me in ways that no other time ever had.

- ❖ As I'm washing dishes, I can hear Mom shuffling through the living room and I peak around the corner to check on her. She comes around the corner with her walker and I ask, "whatcha doin?" She says, "I've been collecting trash for you." Sure enough, the little trash can we keep by her chair is sitting on her walker seat...she had been to the bedroom and bathroom and emptied all the trash cans into one. Looks like I've got myself a helper.

- ❖ Just got Mom settled into bed with a hug and a kiss. She had a funny look on her face, so I said, "Are you all right?" She looked at me very seriously and said, "I'M all right...it's the WORLD!"

- ❖ I just told my mom I was going to go "do something with myself" (ie: hair/make-up). She said, "You're pretty the way you are!" *Moms, never underestimate the power of blessing your daughters with those words...whether they are 5 years old or 51.*

- ❖ A little window into our spa treatment day: I gave Mom a mani/pedi and plucked her chin whiskers *(ladies, don't even try to pretend like you don't know what that's all about!)*. At one point, I said "dang, Mom, plucking your chin is like mowing a lawn with a pair of tweezers!" She was laughing so hard, we had to take a break. We agreed that I wouldn't last one day as an aesthetician *(Mom says "not even one client")*. No tip for me!

- ❖ Awesome quote of the day: Mom was sharing that her father used to say, "You don't like me? I like you just the same." *(Think about it...quite a nice double-meaning way to tell someone to step off.)*

- ❖ I'm helping Mom into her PJ's and she's passing gas a little too close to me for comfort! She sits on the side of the bed, taking a little break, giggling, and says, "Oh Lord, give me the strength to get through this life." I say, "He will, but you might want to ask for forgiveness first!" By now, we're both giggling and she says, "Oh, He understands pressure!"

- ❖ After a delicious taco dinner, a conversation between Mom and my husband: Mom: "That was sooo good, but now I'm stuffed." Mark: "It sure was. I had three. I shouldn't have, but I did."

Just Mom

> Mom: "You ate three? Well...you worked today. *(long pause)* I can't seem to get hired." *(giggles)*

> ❖ Just got Mom all dressed pretty for the day. I said, "There. All set. You look cute!" She responded, "Why thank you! I feel cute!" *See? Even at 87....positive affirmations go a long way for us girls!*

It is my hope that when I share my "Mom-ecdotes" with you, you will find a smile in your heart and also be inspired to journey with your own loved ones on their path. I was ever amazed by her courage, courage that was often propelled by her naughty sense of humor. Mom was very aware that she was battling what the doctors deemed Lewy-Body Dementia. It frustrated and confounded her, but she never allowed it to steal her ability to laugh or to love. She was always watching me, keenly aware of my moods and the fatigue that I tried so hard to hide. No one knows you like your mom and our relationship was no exception. She knew just how to make me smile. One evening, she stared blankly at me as I walked by her chair. Concerned, I stopped in front of her and looked into her eyes. She stared deadpan at me and said, "who are you?" I raised my eyebrow, then seeing the twinkle in her eye, I said, "That's not funny!" She busted out laughing!

> ❖ Mom has gotten really attached to my dog, Bella. She was so distraught yesterday while Bella was at

the vet getting her teeth cleaned, walking around the house saying, "Bella...where are you?" (She knew she was at the vet.) When I brought Bella home, she was still drunk from sedation. Mom felt so bad for her and said, "They can do that kind of thing to dogs, but Bella is not a dog. She's a human!"

- ❖ As Mom was about to stand up, I placed her walker in front of her. She said, "is this curbside service?"

- ❖ Mom is taking her after dinner stroll with her walker through the living room and dining room areas of the house. As she reaches the next room, she mutters, "boy, my get-up-and-go has got up and gone!"

- ❖ Falling stars: Once upon a time, two little twin girls occupied the room that is now my mother's. They covered the ceiling with glow-in-the-dark stars so they could look at them while they were in bed at night. Guess what I found in Mom's bed tonight. (again) *Star light, star bright...*

I remember saying to Mom once how I wished I could just wave a wand and make this horrible disease go away. Her response was an old Scottish proverb, "if wishes were horses, beggars would ride". Indeed, if wishing could make things happen, even the most destitute among us would have all that they wanted. Wishing never helped this journey. Prayer and the knowledge that Jesus walked beside us were the only things that made a difference, and of course, laughter.

- ❖ It's "spa day" for Mom and we just finished with her shower. I told her that her chair in the bedroom (where we do hair, etc) is waiting for her. Her response.."electric?".

- ❖ Mom is so used to me taking pics of her after her "spa day" that, while she was sitting in the chair, naked- with her robe around her shoulders, while I moisturized her, she started chuckling. Then she says, "wanna take a picture now? I look like the Buddha statue!".

- ❖ Sometimes we just need a good hug, and me, being a hugger, sensed that need in my mom tonight. As she sat on the side of her bed, I gave her a big hug and told her that I love her. She said, "I love you, too. No one else would do all the things you do for me." I said, "Aw, yes they would, and I'm not doing anything for you that you haven't already done for me." Then I hear her chuckling into my shoulder as she says, "except you're breaking my nose!"

- ❖ I had a mini-avalanche in my dish drainer while I was washing dishes tonight. Above the clatter, Mom chimes in from the other room, "You're s'pose to break 'em BEFORE you wash 'em!"

- ❖ Mom and I were watching "A Few Good Pie Places" on PBS this afternoon. As we saw pie after pie after delicious pie being savored, Mom said, "there should be a law against programs like this!".

One of the horrible symptoms of Lewy-Body is a chronically runny nose. This plagued Mom terribly. We went through box after box of tissues. Because we also learned that most allergy medications trigger the Lewy Body delusions, there was no easy fix. Each time her tissue box got about ½ inch from the bottom, she would pull all the tissues out and ask for a new box. Then, she would stuff the ones from the old box into the new box. This was usually followed by the story of when my Aunt Myra worked in a tissue factory. My aunt had the same wicked sense of humor as my mom. Apparently, one day, she decided to put a banana peel between the tissues in a box that she was assembling. We often wondered who opened that one up.

- ❖ Mom's allergies are acting up and she had sneezed a few times. I wasn't really paying attention until, through laughter, she said, "How many more times do I have to sneeze before you bless me?!"

- ❖ I'm normally pretty diligent about fixing healthy, balanced meals for Mom. Today she wanted a danish & a cup of tea for lunch. I said, "Is that a healthy lunch choice?" She laughed and said, "No....I'm a JUNKIE!". *We compromised by adding a couple slices of cheddar cheese and a good herbal tea.*

- ❖ Some days are hard and even though we may endeavor to smile through it, parts of the journey just suck. Tonight, as I kissed my mom goodnight, she said, "Thank you for everything you do for me...even when I'm a stinker."

I have come to realize that I have inherited my mom's sense of humor. Somewhere in this journey, as my mom repeatedly mistook me for various other women in our lives, I started hearing Whitney Houston singing, "I'm Every Woman" softly in the background. I've earned my own theme song.

- ❖ Warning: Dark humor. As l was tucking Mom into bed tonight, I asked her if she wanted to be covered up (sometimes the blankets annoy her). She said, "No". Concerned, I said, "Are you sure?

You're cold!". She started chuckling and replied, "No--they refrigerate you at the end anyway!"

- ❖ Mom and I always close our day with a hug and a kiss and an "I love you". Tonight, she asked me how much I love her. My reply was, "To the moon and back." She said, "How about a bushel and a peck? Remember when you used to sing that to Luke (my son) when he was a baby?" Tonight, we closed our day with a sweet song, two spirits loving each other when words aren't adequate. After our song, she said, "I love you more than that."

- ❖ It was nearing her nap time. Mom looked at me and said, "you don't mind if I lie down for a while do you?". I said, "Of course not...you can do anything you want to do." To which she responded, "Can I hug you?".

Sometimes my mom has dreams...dreams so real that, even upon waking, she remains trapped in them. Tonight, was one of those times. I heard her calling out in the fearful tone that I've come to recognize and went immediately to her bedside. It took a long time of repeatedly reminding her of where she was, talking softly to her, gently rubbing her back, anything I could think of to calm her and bring her back. She knew me--she couldn't remember my name, but she knew that I am her daughter. You see, love transcends our memories. So even when we forget words and names, we recognize love. As tears fell softly between us as we sorted through the confusion, I asked her if she would like me to pray for her. She took my hand as though it were a lifeline and said a very firm, "yes!". So, I prayed, and together we entered the presence of Abba God, Daddy, our Comforter, Healer, and Protector—Jesus, our loving High Priest, who knows our hurts and bears our burdens. As I said, "Amen", Mom took up the mantle and offered her own sweet, teary prayer of thanksgiving. We talked a while longer after that and Mom expressed how happy she is that we know Jesus. It occurred to me at that moment that bringing me to Jesus is truly the greatest gift my mom has ever given to me. And tonight, it is a gift we shared equally...a strength and a hope...the very presence of God that will carry us through this valley together.

She had another restless night a few nights later. I awoke in the wee hours of the morning to find her sitting on the side of her bed, completely dressed, bedroom completely dismantled of all of her clothes and belongings, which she had neatly packed up and piled in the middle of the floor. Keep in mind, we are talking about an individual who, on a normal day, couldn't even dress herself. She said "they" told her that she needed to be packed and ready for a trip. (She later told me that "they" were missionaries that she had been on a trip with and was supposed to go on another, but that when I came into the room, the plans were canceled). In a state of utter exhaustion. I told her that there was no trip, that she needed to get back into bed and go to sleep. I put the room back together, put her PJ's back on her, and tucked her into bed. She asked me if she could go to sleep now. I said, "yes, you need to sleep and so do I". She said, "Oh that sounds good to me." We ignored the "baby kittens" that she saw at the end of the bed and the tiny bugs she saw crawling all over the floor. I kissed her on the cheek and told her I love her, which she reciprocated. She slept for 12 hours after that…a truly peaceful sleep with no acting out or talking or grimacing. I prayed that God was "resetting her dial". That's what I called the hours of sleeping that often followed a Lewy episode. It was like a reset. She would wake up as herself again. Hopefully.

After an entire day of sleeping, Mom made her way back from the dark clutches of Lewy-Body. She had a little food and drink and asked me why she is so tired. I explained that she hadn't had much sleep over the last two days due to dreams and delirium. I told her some of the things she had done. She didn't remember any of it. As she digested what I had told her, she looked up at me and, with pained expression asked, "did I hurt anyone?" I assured her that she had not. My mom, who I'd never seen cry, immediately burst into tears...partly from relief and partly from mourning at the realization that this awful disease would continue to steal and plunder.

❖ A couple of days after Mom's "very real" waking dream (delusion) about the 2-week trip with missionaries, I was hanging her freshly laundered clothes in her closet, I said, "hmmm, I'm one hanger short." Mom, back to her quick-humored state, quipped, "That's strange, maybe it's still with the missionaries."

❖ Tonight, was one of those nights when Mom was having trouble remembering my name. At one point, she said, "who are you again?" I smiled and said, "just call me George". She laughed, then I reminded her that I am Beverly. She said, "ah, the last Mohican." *(I'm the baby of the family, hence the name).* Five minutes later, as I kissed her goodnight, she had forgotten again. She said, "Goodnight ____" and I quickly filled in the blank with "George". She was giggling as I again reminded her of my true name. Laughing even harder she said, "Maybe I'll remember in the morning...A-B-C-D..."

Mom and I often talked about how important it is to live in the present. She said, "the good Lord put your eyes on the front of your face for a reason--to look forward". She had an uncanny perspective on the brevity of life and the importance of not only savoring every moment, but also for being thankful for God's blessings TODAY. My dog, Bella, gave me a perfect example of this during a walk.

She kept looking behind us, concerned about whatever may have been back there. The thing that originally piqued her curiosity had long-since gone away, but she still continued to look back. I don't know how many times she ran into my leg or a tree because she was walking forward but looking backward. Yup, eyes in front. Great words, Mom!

- ❖ As I gave Mom a goodnight hug and kiss, she said, "Oh, you're warm!". Next thing I knew, her icy cold hands were in the sleeves of my t-shirt and she was giggling herself silly!

- ❖ After a "not so great" day, I'm tucking my mom into bed and ask, "do you want me to cover you up?" to which she responds, "with dirt?".

- ❖ Today Mom was lamenting about not being able to do the things she used to be able to do. I said, "Well, you can't look back. You have to look forward. My mom told me that's why God put your eyes on the front of your face." She replied, "Well, that woman thinks she knows everything."

- ❖ Mom was trying to kick her slippers off and they ended up flipped around, heels dangling from her toes. She looked at me and said, "I bet you can't do that!"

- Mom asked me for "a mayonnaise sandwich" for lunch. Then she says, "and don't be 'Scotch' on the mayonnaise." *(I was able to talk her into at least having a sliced tomato in that mayo!)*

- Mom was giving me a hug tonight, sympathetic to my stress level due to helping another family member who was having health issues. I told her she's the best mom ever and added, "I don't know how you've put up with all the crap you've had to deal with over the years." She laughed and said, "Well, I've graduated. You haven't graduated yet!"

- In order for my mom to end up high enough on her pillow when I lift her legs into bed at night, she needs to sit in a certain spot on the side of the bed as a starting position. This will be a familiar technique to any of my CNA or nurse friends. It usually takes a couple of tries to get her to scoot down to the right spot. Tonight, she sat down, almost at the right spot, and as usual, I said, "a little bit more". She scooted again, and I said, "one more time". Exhausted and out-of-breath, she dead-pans: "That's what she said!".

- Mom: "I feel dumb today". Me: "dumb?" Mom: "yeah...you know, duhhh?" Me: "Well, you don't seem dumb". Mom: "It's an act."

- Mom was watching the news tonight when they showed a clip of Donald Trump saying that he'd "do a better job than anyone else has ever done" as president. Mom laughed and said, "that wouldn't be too difficult!"

- Mom sneezed and I said, "God bless you!". She said, "Thank you...He'd better do SOMETHING with me!"

- Mom was having a bit of a rough day today. Tonight, as I was tucking her in, I gave her the usual hug and kiss, then said, "I love you". She responded with a disgusted, "I don't know why." I said, "Because you're my mom." She laughed and said, "Well, that's a good reason...I love you, too, *Barb*." (sigh...Lewy can't steal the love!!)

- Trying to explain to my mom what hummus is, l tell her it's mashed up beans, and she immediately says, "instead of real farts, they hummm?"

- Watching ice skating on TV with Mom. As the male skater lifts his female partner over his shoulders, Mom says, "I hope she has good life insurance."

- I lean down to kiss her goodnight and she puts one icy hand on each side of my neck. I say, "this is not about love...you're just trying to steal my body heat!" She was laughing so hard; she couldn't even speak.

- ❖ Lunchtime discussion with Mom:
  Mom: I'll have a cup of tea and a piece of key lime pie.
  Me: That's not healthy.
  Mom: I don't care.

- ❖ Mom has a love / hate relationship with her mattress. Tonight, it's the latter. She told me that hard mattresses are better for you (as opposed to the pillowtop that she currently has). I was trying to explain that hard mattresses are actually worse due to pressure points, etc. She looked at me, fluttered her eyelashes and, in her best "fancy, Southern lady" accent, said, "well I don't know what this is, but I don't liiiike it."

- ❖ I bend down to kiss Mom goodnight and she reaches up with her icy-cold hands and says, "let me touch this hot mama!" *I told her she's getting mittens for Christmas.*

- ❖ Returning to the living room after helping mom in the bathroom, she pushes by with her walker (which has a seat) and says, "Want a ride or are you walking back?"

❖ I just gave Mom her dinner and asked her how it is. She said, "It's delicious!" Then, "I'm afraid I'll have to stay!"

❖ Mom was so cute this afternoon. She took a long nap after "Spa-Day", as usual. First words out of her mouth when she woke up? "Oh, I bet I messed my hair all up!". *Girls still want to be pretty...even at 88.*

SIX MONTHS IN
A NEW YEAR

As we turned the page on the calendar to a new year, it wasn't lost on me that Mom had already outlived the doctor's prognosis. According to him, she was healthier than ever. He was astounded at her progress. There is something to be said for good food and a loving, peaceful environment.

- ❖ As she opens her arms so I can help her with her sweater, she pulls me into a hug and says, "Ooo I knew I'd get you." Yes, Mom, you've got me...and I've got you, too.

- ❖ As I help Mom out of the shower and into her warm robe, she starts singing, "Baby, it's cold outside...".

- ❖ Laughing so hard right now. I'm watching Kathie Lee & Hoda with Mom. Jenna Bush is sitting in for Kathie Lee today. We love Jenna. Out of the blue, Mom says, "They never show her twin, do they...*(wait for it)*...is she ugly or what?" *(our apologies to Barbara. lol)*

- ❖ Watching TV with Mom and a commercial for Amish Cleaning Tonic came on touting its household cleaning power. Mom says, "Fooey on the Cleaning Tonic! I want someone to come *do* the cleaning for me!"

❖ Yesterday: "Why is your face yellow?" Today: "Boy, you've really gone gray!" *Why, thank you, Mom! Good thing this jaundiced, silver-haired mare has a sense of humor!*

❖ Mom was coughing a few minutes ago (probably a result of today's drier air) and I teasingly said, "You been smoking again? I told you to quit that!" Without missing a beat, she replied, "You told me to quit smoking, but you didn't say anything about using snuff!"

❖ Mom has some of the brain/body "disconnect" issues that are characteristic of Lewy-Body. It's worse when she is fatigued. Tonight, as she was walking to her bed, one leg wasn't listening very well, causing her gait to be a bit off. She chuckled and said, "My father had a horse that walked like this!"

❖ At the doctor with mom. The tech was having trouble getting a blood pressure reading with the automatic reader. She turns to mom and says, "I'm going to use the manual reader--don't want you to get mad at me for blowing you up over and over with this thing". Mom looks at her and says, "Only dogs get mad".

- Mom just looked at me and said, "You're pretty". I smiled and said, "aww, well thank you. YOU'RE pretty!". She laughed and said, "pretty OLD!". *She's always gotta have the last word.*

- Mom's hip has been bothering her the last couple of days. She turned to me as she was slowly getting up from her chair and said, "I sure would like to know who did this to my hip." I jokingly said, "Well, if you'd quit sneaking out at night, carousing with men we don't know..." She laughed and said, "That'll do it!"... then in a serious tone, not sure what Lewy may have had her up to, "Do I do that?". *No, Mom. I'm just teasing you.*

- I was doing Mom's hair and had just sprayed some hairspray to hold her 'do in place when she said, "Will you spray some of that on my back? Maybe it will straighten it out."

- I noticed Mom starting to doze in the chair and said, "Are you falling asleep?". She replied, "No, my eyes were."

- Mom, as she heads in for a nap: "Hello, bed. Are you ready for me?" *(I, of course, hear Adele singing softly in the background. "Hello...")*

Just Mom

- ❖ I just mentioned to Mom that the color blue is an appetite suppressant and that it's supposed to help with weight loss to eat on a blue plate. She thought about it for a second and said, "I guess there's not enough blue on your plates!"

- ❖ As I was putting Mom to bed, she began to cough. I said, "Do you need a drink?" She stopped coughing, looked at me for a second and said with a giggle, "What are you offering?" *party at Mom's crib tonight!*

- ❖ Mom: "I keep forgetting." Me: "That's what you've got me for!" Mom: "I got you because I wanted you." *Same here, Mom. Same here.*

- ❖ When I asked Mom what she'd like for lunch, she thought about it for a minute and said, "How about just half of a peanut butter sandwich? Just a half though. I haven't worked very hard today."

For many years now, even before she came to live with us, when Mom has had moments of frustration with herself, she'd say, "I hate me". Today we were discussing our various physical issues and she said, "Maybe now you know what I mean when I say, "I hate me". I said that while I do understand what she means, I personally believe that that particular phrase is a slap in the face to

God because we are His special creations that He loves so much. She was quiet for a few moments then she said, "Hmm I never thought of it like that. That's the last time you'll hear that out of my mouth....and I agree with you."

Mom's memory of days gone by was clear as a bell. Interestingly enough, even many of her delusions were centered around towns where she grew up and people whom she used to spend time with as a young person. Apart from the delusions, it was always interesting to hear her reminisce about her childhood.

- ❖ Babies come from doctor's black bags...did you know that? Mom said that when she was just a little girl, one of her older sisters gave birth to a son. Mom said she was running around, brimming with childish excitement about the big event. Her sister's doctor looked down at her and told her to settle down or he would put her back in his black bag. From that time forth, she thought that was where babies came from.

- ❖ It's late afternoon. This is Mom's favorite part of the day when the sun shines through the window onto her chair. We call it her "vitamin D therapy". So, I'm in the kitchen making dinner and she calls to me and says, "I've got some broiled brain here, if you want some...broiled by the sun!" It's a dark humor kind of day.

- ❖ Tonight, I gave Mom a kiss goodnight as I tucked her into bed and said, "I love you." She said, "I don't know why. I'm such a pain." I frowned at her and said, "Have I ever said that?" She said, "Said what?" I responded, "That you're a pain." She started giggling and said, "You just did! ...Gotcha!" Followed by more laughter.

I've been told frequently throughout my life that I look like my mother. There's no denying that I'm her daughter, that is for sure. Sometimes I see her in my mirror. It's funny how precious inherited characteristics become when we no longer have our people with us.

- ❖ As I situate Mom in a chair directly in front of me in order to perform some aesthetician needs, she looks right into my eyes and starts laughing, saying, "It's like looking in a mirror!" I laugh along with her and say, "Yeah? Welcome to your younger self! How do you like it?" She looks at me approvingly and says, "I like it!"

- ❖ As Mom slowly shuffles by me, heading for a nap, she laments, "this motor don't run right."

- We were watching Raw Travel on TV a little while ago. One of the destinations was a "Hemp" farm in Colorado. Mom watched intently throughout the episode. About an hour later, a random musing from Mom: "Boy, all those acres of marijuana were really beautiful."

- As I get Mom all tucked into bed, she looks up at me with the silliest glimmer in her eyes and says, "My back is broken". I look into her eyes and say, "You're a goofball". She responds with a giggle, "I'm all yours, Sweetie".

- Mom: I'm sorry I called you *Alex.*
  Me: That's okay. I know you know who I am.
  Mom: I should. I gave birth to you.
  Me: Then I guess you can call me anything you want!
  Mom: I like Becky...Rebekah. (my daughter's name) *Cue the "I'm Every Woman" theme song.*

- As I tucked her cozy blanket around her, I said, "Have a nice nap, Mom. I love you." She drowsily responded, "I love you, too...for all you do for me...and a lot of other reasons, too."

- As I'm heading out to walk Bella after getting Mom settled in her chair, I say, "I'm going to walk

Bella. Are you ok for a few minutes?" Mom responds, "I'm ok--a little nutty, but I'm ok."

- ❖ Mom just shuffled by me and said, "Boy, I feel 90 today--that used to be a joke!"

- ❖ As Mom pushes herself out of a chair with a grunt, she laments, "Boy, she weighs a ton!"

- ❖ On the eve of my birthday, as I tuck my mom into bed, say goodnight and tell her that I love her, she kisses me on the cheek and says, "Goodnight, Bev, I love you, too", then adds, "You're gonna be an old gal tomorrow. I was an old gal when I had you!". *(She was 36).* I said, "I know. I'm glad I had my kids at a young age. I don't know how you did it." Her response? "Verrry carefully!"

Mom had overcome many obstacles in her own life and always seemed to hold special compassion for those going through tough times. She was always ready to help someone in need, never asking for anything in return, and never speaking about it again. She would say, "If you give someone something, let go of it". She had a tough exterior that held a heart of gold.

- ❖ Watching tonight's rather dismal newscast with Mom when she says, "Everyone has problems, but not everyone knows how to cope."

- After I got Mom all dressed and hair coiffed, I gave her a hug and said, "Ok, off you go!". She responded with a hearty musical, "into the wild, blue yonder..."

- As the afternoon sun begins to pour through the window by Mom's chair, she reclines a little further and I say, "Ohhh your sun shower is happening!" She responds with, "I know. I have a reservation."

- As I was doing Mom's hair this morning after her relaxing shower, her head kept falling forward. As I gently pushed it back (again), she chuckled and said, "That hinge is broken!"

- As we're watching "Wheel" tonight, I lazily recline back on the sofa in a fairly pretzel-like fashion. Mom glances at me and says, "That's not a very lady-like position." I wiggled my eyebrows at her and said, "I'm no lady." *She's still chuckling.*

- Heading to Publix while my husband sits with Mom. On the way out the door, I say, "You two behave yourselves. I'll be right back." Mom looks blankly at me, so I say, "Did you hear me, Mom? No wild parties." Without missing a beat, she deadpans, "You're the one that's on the loose."

- Mom keeps pushing the forward and backwards buttons on her electric recliner. I look at her and say, "Is it kind of like a Fair ride?" She snickers and says, "Yeah...wanna try it?"

- Mom, watching a commercial on TV: "He's had that same shirt on for the last week."

- I was complaining about the hot weather to Mom and how long it takes my body to get cooled back down after being outside. I laughed and said, "I think I'm getting old!" She furrowed her brow and said, "half a hundred!"

- Mom was watching a commercial for a local kitchen remodeling company that has their whole, huge family in it. The patriarch of the family was talking about how much time they spend with their customers in order to create their dream kitchen. Mom looked intently at the screen and said in a rather disgusted voice, "I think they spent a lot of time in the bedroom!"

- Mom looked at my outfit today and said, "That's nice. I like that." She seems to look forward to seeing what I throw on each day and usually has something to say about it. I thanked her for the compliment, then she said, "I love your clothes!"

Some things truly never change...8 or 88...girls will be girls!

❖ Mom, dozing on and off in her chair: "Somebody keeps closing my eyes!"

Mom's back is bothering her today. As she was making her way to her room tonight, she started "folding in half". She said, in a panic, "I'm going down!" I was walking behind her, as usual, and placed my arms around her, straightening her against my body, telling her, "I will be your back brace." She thanked me, then said, "Somebody rubbed some stuff on me earlier. Was that you?". "Yes, that was me." And then, "Will you do that again?" *Dear Lewy-Body Dementia: I despise you.*

❖ Mom and I were watching The Dog Whisperer and I said, "I prefer medium-sized dogs. Bella is considered a medium-sized dog." Mom looked at me and said, "Bella is considered a human being!"

❖ Mom: "I would like to zip around but my zipper's broken."

❖ They just modeled "sailor-inspired" pants (with the two rows of buttons) on TV. Mom said, "we used to have a joke...'why do sailors have all those buttons on their pants?'" I said, "why?" She smiled and responded, "to give them a chance to change their minds."

Mom is keenly aware of the sacrificial life of a caregiver. As I was dressing her this morning, she looked up at me and asked, "What would you be doing if you didn't have me?" The question caught me totally off guard. My immediate response was that it doesn't matter. I work very hard to remain in the moment rather than looking over the fence. That said, it set my mind to spinning. What would I be doing? Lunches with friends? Interacting more in the community? Travel? Longer walks? Date nights with my hubby? Random daily escapes by car or boat? Yes. All of those things...but after the flutter of activity quieted in my brain, I found the true answer to Mom's question. What would I be doing if I didn't have her? *"Nothing as important as this."*

- ❖ I kissed Mom goodnight and said, "I love you." With a twinkle in her eye, she responded, "I loved you first."

- ❖ On the phone with an insurance rep getting Mom's mailing address updated (one I overlooked after we moved her to our home). The Rep, needing to have Mom verbally verify my relationship to her, asks her my name. Mom, drawing a blank, looks at me and says, "Who are you?" I just look at her as she asks me to tell her my name, then, realizing that she's serious, I say, "Beverly". *Momma never said there'd be days like this.*

In an effort to add a little more cognitive stimulation to Mom's world, I decided to make a puzzle area in our living room. I went out and bought a 1,000-piece puzzle depicting a lakeside cabin, then rearranged my living room to create a puzzle area. Mom then informed me that she doesn't like doing puzzles. She does seem to enjoy watching me do puzzles, though. I don't enjoy doing puzzles either, but my OCD-ness won't allow me to leave it undone. Guess who's getting her cognitive work-out on in her new puzzle area? Hint: It's not Mom! Did I mention that Mom told me that I said my first swear word at the age of three *while doing a puzzle?*

- ❖ Did the "spa day" routine with Mom this morning. Later, after her nap, I was serving her lunch and told her that her hair looks pretty. She looked up at me and said, "That's my daughter's hair." *(because I'm also her hair dresser).*

- ❖ There was a Macaw on the Today Show this morning that sparked a memory for Mom. She said, "My father used to have a parrot. He taught it to say, "Polly want a cracker? Crack 'er yourself, you brought her here!"

Just Mom

- ❖ I took Bella for a nail trim this afternoon and now she's conked out next to me on the sofa. Mom is half-dozing in her chair nearby. I said, "my poor little dog is all worn out now". Mom looked over at us and said, "That's the way us old dogs are!"

- ❖ Mom holds her hand out to me and says, "look at my hand". I say, "what's the matter with it?". As she lifts the other one up, she responds, "all wrinkled...look at this one!"

- ❖ Mom just shuffled by with her walker, bumping into the corner of the coffee table as she went. Under her breath she says, "Drunk driver."

- ❖ Watching Wheel of Fortune with Mom. I solved the final puzzle. The show ended. Mom turned to me and said, "Go get your money!"

Things that make you go "hmmm": What if dementia isn't so much a disease as it is the thinning of a veil between this reality and another? As my mother is up before dawn, wandering in confusion, I ask her what she's doing. She doesn't know. I say, "You're at Mark and Bev's." Still confused, she responds, "I know, but everything's different." Placing my arm around her, I say, "Let's go back to bed. You're just confused. You'll feel better later when you wake up." *(PS. I do not like this version of reality.)* And just to reinforce my point, later in the afternoon, when Mom was closing her eyes for a nap, she said, "ok, let's see where I can go now." *hmmmm*

- ❖ Mom, just up from her nap, "It's funny how far you can go in a short length of time."

- ❖ Mom, watching a brief news clip about Trump and Clinton: "I swear Bella is smarter than both of them."

- ❖ As I'm rubbing moisturizer on Mom's legs this morning, she says, "Rub some of this fat off while you're at it!"

- ❖ Mom, during our bathing/dressing ritual: "Aren't you glad babies don't come this big?"

- ❖ As Mom shuffles toward her bed in Tim Conway's "old man" style, she pauses for a moment, looks up at it and says with an exhausted voice, "Get ready, bed. Here I come!"

- ❖ Watching Jeopardy with Mom, and on this rare occasion, I was actually able to answer some questions. I turn to Mom and jokingly say, "Hey, Mom, I won some money!" She dryly responds with, "Don't spend it all in one place."

Just Mom

One of the banes of my mom's existence throughout her final years was her mattress, actually every mattress. She had been uncomfortable on her mattress at her house and had intended to replace it prior to all of this happening. She never got that opportunity. She complained about the mattress at the rehabilitation center. I bought a memory foam topper for that one which she promptly had me remove. When she moved in with us, she complained about the relatively new, guestroom mattress that had become her new bed. We then bought a brand new, top of the line mattress for her. She liked it for approximately one week. It was, after that time, forever referred to at "that damn mattress". She insisted that it was *used* and that the company had pulled a fast one on me. I began to realize, because there were times that she was, indeed, quite comfortable, that the problem was not the mattress, nor was it ever. The problem was Lewy.

- ❖ "I have to get in just the right spot where whoever had this mattress before me has left a hole."

- ❖ Mom, struggling to keep her head upright as I comb her hair, "How much does the human head weigh?" *(The answer is "about 11 pounds" in case you're interested.)*

- ❖ As I wrap the shower turban around Mom's head after her bath, she says, "Got my brain all packed in there?" "Yup, right in your 11-pound head."

❖ There was a commercial on for some drug, and the announcer began rattling off all the side effects in rapid succession. All of a sudden, I hear Mom saying, "blablablablablalalala..." Guess that's what it sounded like to her.

❖ Me: "Good morning. You're up early today." Mom: "Well, someone opened my door." *Nope.*

❖ Mom is telling me about the crazy dream/hallucinations that she had in the wee hours of the morning and upon waking this morning. Suddenly she puts her hands up, and with exasperation says, "I just need to quit drinkin'!"

❖ I'm sitting here coughing with a bout of bronchitis and Mom says, "Did Hillary give that to you?" *Remember Hillary's bronchitis during the campaign?*

During the years with that Mom lived with me, my brother phoned her at a set time almost every morning. Mom would eagerly await those phone calls. She never stopped being our mom. She never stopped caring or needing to know that we were ok. Even at her last, her most pressing thoughts were for our wellbeing. This is something to remember if you have an aging parent, whether they have dementia or not, especially mothers.

Just Mom

Moms never stop being moms, never stop needing to be needed.

- ❖ Mom is having a sleepy day today, with lots of napping. My brother phoned and I overhear him asking her if she's feeling ok. She responded with, "Yeah. I'm ok. I'm just on vacation!"

- ❖ Mom: *(After I make breakfast, dress her, change her sheets, rotate the "damn mattress", sweep her floor, and walk Bella twice, all while fighting the flu, which I've apparently concealed well...)* "I feel bad for the people who have to keep working when they're sick."

- ❖ Best reward for pushing my sick self through the "spa day" ritual? Seeing my Mom looking so fresh, pretty, and relaxed...getting a hug and being told, "I love you. You're the greatest."

- ❖ Mom, as we're discussing the flu that's going around: "Yours is much better than it was." Me: "No, it isn't much better." Mom: "Well, that's your opinion."

- ❖ Mom, walking from bathroom to bedroom where I was waiting to dress her for the day, didn't bother to pull her PJ bottoms all the way back up; "My pants are half down. I'd fit right in with some of these young people today."

❖ There is a woman on TV whose hair is bleached blond and cropped very short. Mom, in the process of standing up, looks very intently at her and says, "What is that on her head?". I laugh and say, "Mom, that's her hair!" She responds by furrowing her brow, shaking her head, and shuffling off with her walker.

❖ I was telling Mom what a nice vacation taking a cruise is. I said, "It's so relaxing. Everything is done for you." She thought for a moment, then asked, "What's the name of *this* cruise?"

❖ Mom takes a little walk with the assistance of her walker, around the living/dining area and back to her chair. She parks her walker and sits down with a sigh. I ask her if she's ok and she says, "I don't know." I ask for clarity. She says, "I'm not ok mentally." I say, "What does that mean?" She responds with a dark chuckle, "I just can't get my sh*t together!"

Awaking to Mom screaming with delirium was jolting, to say the least, but far worse were the times that I was awakened by a "thud", knowing that she had fallen. My heart would lurch. I would leap out of bed, yelling to my

Just Mom

husband to wake up, and the two of us would rush to her room or hallway or bathroom to assess the situation. I lost track of the number of times that we had to pick her up. It was a miracle that she was never seriously injured. Mom was not a petite lady. She and I used to laugh about the benefits of having a little extra "padding" on our bones; God's crash protection.

- ❖ Mom, fell in the night while returning to her room from the bathroom. She was attempting to shut her bedroom door and lost her balance, landing in a sitting position against the wall. No breaks or bruises, but a sore tailbone. She said she has "what you would call a pain in the ass."

- ❖ Mom, on the phone with my cousin: "I fell the other night." Cousin: "You did? What happened?!" Mom, not missing a beat, "Too much liquor."

- ❖ I'm giving Mom her shower and have her all lathered up with soap. She starts to chuckle. I ask her what she's laughing at. She says, "I look like a snowman!" *Merry Christmas!*

- ❖ Mom was up a bit early this morning. Me: "Good morning. You're up and at 'em this morning!" Mom: "I couldn't lay there any longer." *Ten minutes later, asleep in her chair....and an extra cup of coffee for me!*

Many years ago, I found out that I have a gluten allergy. I have been gluten-free ever since. When Mom came to live with us, I followed a similar eating plan for her. I credit "clean eating", at least in part, with the extra years that she was able to live past the doctor's initial projection, as well as the relative stability of her disease during that time. Each morning, she enjoyed a gluten-free blueberry waffle and yogurt with fresh fruit, along with coffee and juice. She looked forward to her breakfast every single day and rarely wanted anything different.

- ❖ Mom and I usually have gluten-free blueberry waffles for breakfast. She has fresh fruit & yogurt on the side. I slather mine with peanut butter. *(Don't judge).* Today I only had one gluten-free waffle, so I substituted a regular waffle for Mom, thinking she wouldn't notice. Mom took one bite of her waffle and said, "these waffles aren't as good as the other ones!"

My favorite times with Mom were the sweet, oftentimes hilariously funny, conversations that took place as I was putting her to bed. Sometimes we would laugh till we cried, other times, she would touch my heart with the most loving, heartfelt sentiments. She had never been one to be "mushy" with her words, but Lewy changed all of that. She didn't hold back during her final years. It was as though she needed me to know how she felt, needed me to hold onto her thoughts for her. They will reside in the jewel box of my heart forever.

- ❖ Tonight's pillow talk: I got Mom all tucked into bed and she said, "I love you." I responded, "I love you, too." She, exasperated with her limitations, said, "I don't know why." I said, "Well, why do *you* love *me*?" She raised her eyebrows and responded, "Because you're my baby!" I laughed and said, "Well, *you're* my *mother, so, there!*" She chuckled and said, "Okay. Score one!"

- ❖ Mom's random, profound morning comment as she watches the news on television: "I wouldn't want to be young again." I ask, "Why is that?" She deadpans, "Because I think our world is nuts!"

- ❖ I ask Mom what she'd like for lunch and start listing options. She says, "How 'bout ice cream?" I laugh and say, "I don't think that's very healthy." She furrows her brow and responds, "What difference does it make if it's healthy?"

- ❖ Mom told me that I need to put a red ribbon around Bella's neck. When I asked her why, she said, "to show that she's a Republican!" *(I think Bella is Libertarian, FYI)*

- Mom has a habit of sitting a little catawampus in her chair, then needing help to readjust. After I helped her into her chair just now, I said, "are you straight?" She thought for a moment and said, "I haven't even been out!"

- As I was tucking Mom in tonight, she said, "I love you. It's been a nice day." *What more can a person ask for?*

- Mom: "Hollie, (my daughter who is a photographer) is always taking wedding pictures. Does she ever take any *divorce* pictures?"

- Watching Wheel of Fortune with Mom and I say, "I like Vanna's dress." Mom says, "Tell her to send it over." I say, "I don't think I'll have any more occasions where I'll need to dress that fancy now that the kids are all married." Mom thinks for a second, then quips, "You never know, I might find some rich old man!"

- My husband, walking toward our bedroom: "Well, I'm gonna go take a shower." Mom: "Ya want me to wash your back?"

- Mom requested carrot cake for her birthday tomorrow, so I whipped up a batch of (gluten-free) carrot cake cupcakes. Mom watched every step of the process *(kind of like a hawk watching its prey)*. After I got them all arranged and decorated, there were a couple leftover that didn't fit in the arrangement. I asked Mom if she wanted a sample. She, very excitedly, said, "YES!" I gave her one and she was like a kid, enjoying every bite. After the last bite, she licked her lips and said, "Boy! I'm glad I lived to be 89!" *(Me, too, Mom.)*

❖ Heading out the door to walk Bella, I say to Mom, "I'll be right back." She laughs a mischievous laugh and says, "I'll be eating cupcakes!"

❖ Mom has had such a nice birthday, receiving visits, gifts, phone calls, and internet greetings. Tonight, as she got up from her chair to head to bed, she was visibly tired from the festivities of the day. She stood there in front of her chair, holding onto her walker, not moving. I looked at her. She looked at me. Then, with the tiniest twinkle in her eye, she said, "Make this thing go, will you?"

❖ Just a day after her birthday, Mom, a meticulous organizer, removed a handful of birthday cards and photos from the little table next to her chair. She asked me if I had a box to put them in. I understood her taking her birthday cards down *(even though I tend to leave mine up for a week after my birthday),* but the photos baffled me. They were pictures of her kids and grandkids, displayed in a photo stand. I said, "Did you mean to take the photos down, too?" Her response was, "Yeah. I know what they look like!" *Lewy has a dark side.*

One of the most frustrating symptoms of Lewy-Body Dementia is it's paring with Parkinson's. Mom developed a tremor in her leg that often had a mind of its own. She called it her "dancing leg".

- ❖ Mom just got up from her nap and, as I was helping her into her chair (which entails supporting her arm as she toddles the two feet from where she parks her walker, then waiting while her 'dancing leg' simmers down so she can sit, then adjusting her back pillow once she gets her bod in place) she sighs and says, "that damn Ruth!"

- ❖ We bought Mom a new sweater for Christmas. When I put it on her this morning, I said, "how's that feel?" She gave me a hug and said, "It feels like you, nice and soft."

- ❖ Mom, watching the news on tv: "Some of these homely people make *me* feel good."

THE MONSTER CALLED LEWY-BODY

I've told you many funny stories about my mom's days with us, how her cheeky sense of humor made me giggle or how we both laughed so hard at something inappropriate that we nearly lost our breath.

There were things that were not at all funny, though, things I haven't told you, like the fact that when she called me by other people's names, it was often not a slip of the tongue, but because she truly thought I *was* someone else. There were the many times I saw her looking really hard at me the way you look at someone you know you know, but just can't place. Once, during a lucid time, I asked her where I, *Beverly*, go when she sees me as someone else. She said, "I don't know. You're just not here." There was also that time when she looked at me and said, "I know this is a strange question, but what year did you move to Florida?" And after discussing the fact that I moved here with her and my dad and brother when I was 5 years old, she said, "so you grew up here." She misplaced me so many times.

In order for me to stay present and not lost in grief, I did something I never thought I'd do. I had a tattoo put on my wrist in my Mom's handwriting that simply says, "Love" with roots leading down to a heart to remind me that even though Lewy stole my identity in my Mom's brain, it could never ever steal the love that we shared. It helped me through many rough days. It still does. Don't ever judge someone with tattoos. You may not know their story. Ask. They will probably tell you.

I didn't tell you that she often thought I rearranged the house while she napped. She would wake up, enter the living room, swear that I had changed it all around, and get angry when I promised that I didn't.

I didn't tell you how many times I held her in my arms, soothing her as she wept, body wracked with mourning, whenever the truth of her Lewy-Body would resurface and she realized that she was losing the battle.

I didn't mention the day that she asked me to look behind her as she pointed to her back because *"it feels like a piece of me is missing"*. That was the best description of Lewy-Body's thievery that I've ever heard.

She saw children in her bed almost nightly or her deceased siblings in her room or strangers wandering about the house or car lights shining in her bedroom window at night, or a man whistling outside. She would ask me about them, only to realize with futility, that they were visible to her alone.

She never stopped teaching me. Like, when she asked me what was happening to her and we had a talk about Lewy-Body Dementia…and she said, "oh well, as long as I don't have to be in pain..." *Acceptance. Trust. Grace. Strength.*

I didn't tell you how she lamented not being given time to organize things in her condo before dementia started to take from her. *Seize the day.*

There were numerous times that she asked me if she was ever going to get better "than she is right now" and I had to answer her, "no". *Honesty.*

There were times when she asked me, "when will I go to sleep and not wake up?", and I had to remind her that only God knows the answer to that question. *Faith. Endurance.*

So often, her Lewy-Body confusion was literally like watching a TV station that couldn't seem to stay on one channel but constantly had interference from other channels, and during the few times that the channel got "dialed in", she would ask me very frank questions about her disease, through *uncontrollable tears* "Is this *(the crying)* all part of what I've got going on?" *Yes.*

I did my best to preserve her dignity while performing the most intimate of tasks. There were times when I was helping her with her bathroom needs and she would say, "I'll be glad when you don't have to do this for me anymore." I would try to keep from tearing up, because I knew that that would mean she would no longer be with us.

I never shared the breaking of my heart as our roles became completely reversed and she began to call me, "Mom".

I didn't say how privileged I was... how grateful I *am* that my amazing, strong, independent mother chose to *allow* me to care for her, to hold her hand and walk with her through the Valley of the Shadow. Lewy-Body took my mom, but it can never have what she has given me.

Beverly Carriere Tiner

THE SECOND YEAR

Just Mom

As the journey became more difficult during the third year, and Mom's physical needs became greater, I realized that I needed help. I was blessed with a few incredible, private duty aides. At first, I hired them for a couple of days a week for a few hours at a time. It allowed me some self-care that I desperately needed and it gave Mom a bit of interaction besides that of myself or my husband. She called them her "babysitters". She grew very attached to them, and they to her. In the end, I believe she may have given them an even greater gift than they gave her. For me, though, they became a life-line.

- ❖ Watching Jeopardy with Mom. It's a rare night and I'm actually answering a string of questions. After I answered the last one, Mom pipes up and says, "You know you're not gonna win nothin'...?"

- ❖ The answer to one of the Jeopardy questions involved Dover, the capital of Delaware. Suddenly Mom says, "What did Dela-wear? I don't know...Al-ask-ah."

- ❖ Mom's navigating a little slow today. As she shuffles across the living room, bumping her walker on the corner of the coffee table, she says, "My legs don't wanna walk." I say, "Well, if you'd quit drinkin', you'd be alright." She chuckles and says, "I never thought of that."

❖ We took Mom for routine bloodwork this morning. As she was watching the crazy drivers on the highway zoom by us, Mom says, "We have a driver's license, what the hell do you people have?!"

Valentine's Day is my favorite of all holidays, largely due to the way in which my mom celebrated it. Throughout most of my growing-up years, it would be on Valentine's Day morning that I would awake to a sweet little gift left upon my dresser. My mom, a woman who rarely expressed loving sentiments verbally, chose that day each year to tell me how very much she loved me.

❖ It's Valentine's Day. As I lean down in front of her to do up the snaps on her robe after today's shower, a kiss is placed softly on the side of my neck. No words needed. She'll always be my first Valentine.

❖ Mom just stretched, and in a sing-song, kind of exasperated voice, went "oh ho ho ho". I said, "that bad?". She snickered and replied, "that GOOD!".

❖ I'm wearing one of those "cold-shoulder" shirts today. Mom made a point this morning to tell me that she liked my outfit. Later, she looked intently at my sleeve and said, "your blouse is torn".

- ❖ I had just come from my bedroom after getting dressed, and was then in Mom's room, dressing her. She asked me if I was ok and I responded that I had gotten really hot when I was in my bedroom. She chuckled and said, "Well, that's the place to get hot!"

- ❖ Me: "What would you like for lunch?" Mom: "I'll have a banana split." ...*and a banana split she did have!* Hearing her "mmm that's good" after the first few bites is all the proof needed that we should indulge ourselves on occasion. I hope that, if I live to be 89, someone will indulge me with inappropriate food as well! *Hear that, kids?*

- ❖ Mom: "My words get lost." Me: "It's ok. It happens." Mom: "Well, it's crap."

- ❖ As I'm tucking Mom into bed, she looks kind of expressionless at the ceiling. I lean close to her face and pull her covers up around her shoulders. As I glance at her face, she suddenly jerks in my direction and goes, "BOO!". *Dear God, woman!*

- ❖ I asked Mom if she wanted me to take a "Spa Day" picture today. She's all relaxed with hair freshly done. Apparently, she's REALLY relaxed, because her response was, "No, I feel like a zombie."

- ❖ I was helping Mom roll her walker over the thresholds at the bathroom/bedroom doorways tonight as it's more difficult for her when she's tired. I gave one wheel a little nudge to help her along and she said, "You drive better than I do!"

I came to dread the full moon each month. While there is, apparently no scientific proof of its affect, Mom would have an "episode" every full moon. It usually started early in the day with glitchy moments of confusion, culminating with a night filled with dreams and delusions, often lasting up to 48 hours.

- ❖ Mom's been having what I call a "glitchy" day today, as often happens with a pending full moon. She has called me by one of my sister's names several times. Tonight, after I tucked her in, she said, "Goodnight, Jean". I just looked at her, waiting to see if she would catch herself. Without missing a beat, she followed up with, "Tell Bev I said goodnight, too." Our "I love you's" were mottled with chuckling as I closed her door.

- ❖ We just finished my delicious birthday dinner with part of my clan. I said, "That was a really nice little celebration." Mom responded, "Yah, I hope when I get that old, you'll do that for me."

Just Mom

- ❖ Mom woke up a little confused this morning, thinking she was somewhere else for a few minutes. Her confusion cleared up pretty quickly once our normal routine resumed. After taking the last bite of her favorite breakfast, she said, "Ahhh I'm glad I was HERE!" *(Blueberry waffles fix everything!)*

- ❖ I said to Mom, "If it's going to be gloomy out, I wish it would rain." She replied, "Well, if wishes were fishes, we'd have an ocean-full."

- ❖ As I'm dressing Mom for bed tonight, she snickers and says, "Hurry up. I'm falling asleep."

- ❖ After getting Mom all dressed and pretty for the day, I said, "Ok, I'm going to go do *me* now." She said, "going to get beautiful?" I laughed and responded, "gonna do *something* anyway!" She smiled and said, "I like you just the way you are."

As Lewy-Body progresses, so does the accompanying fatigue. Mom was no exception to this and it frustrated her greatly. She was once one of the most energetic people I've ever known, always able to run circles around me.

- ❖ Mom just got up from her nap and I asked her if she had a good nap. She said, "yeah, but I just can't figure out why I'm so tired all the time." I waited a few seconds, and instead of giving her some serious answer, I responded, "Well...you're *old!"* Caught off guard, she cracked up, laughing. *Sometimes, you just have to laugh at life.*

- ❖ After the whole "spa day" ritual, I tuck Mom in for her nap, tell her I love her, and she says, "I love you, too, Bev...and all you do for me...you were mine before I was yours."

- ❖ Mom *(watching a cooking show)*: "I wonder who ever thought up eating meat." Me: "Probably Adam and Eve." Mom: I wonder if they ever thought of cutting a human being up and eating them." Me: "Mom! Ewwwwww!!"

- ❖ I'm wearing flowered, camo-green pants and a green shirt today. Mom says: "That looks nice together......got your rifle?"

Today is the 2-year mark since I brought Mom home from the Rehab Hospital to live with us. They told me I should move her to the nursing facility wing. They said it would be too much to care for her at home. The doctor gave her about 6 months. Two years later, she is still with us. It's not a cake-walk, and each day does indeed bring challenges, but oh, the blessings! I would do it again in a

Just Mom

heartbeat. Don't hesitate if you have the desire to bring your elder loved one home. There is assistance available. You don't have to go it alone.

- ❖ As I put Mom to bed and say goodnight, she tells me goodnight but calls me by the wrong name. I look at her for a minute, waiting to see if she notices her mistake. She says, "oh honestly. You are *Beverly*." We both laugh and again I tell her "goodnight" and "I love you". She says, "I love you, too, Honey. I'm just gonna call you *Honey* from now on."

- ❖ As I took Mom's dinner plate from her tonight, I said, "was it good?" She responded, "I didn't like the potato salad." I looked at her quizzically and said, "Mom, that was a baked potato." She scowled and said *a little more firmly,* "well, I didn't like it!"

- ❖ Mom woke up from her afternoon nap a little while ago and just finished having a snack. Suddenly she says, "Boy, all that sleep made me tired!"

A little window into one of our mornings: Mom and I were discussing the ages of various family members. I said, "We're all getting old, Mom!" She said, "I'm not 'getting'. I'm good for nothing at this point." In reminding her that she still has a purpose on this earth, I told her that every person with whom she comes into contact can benefit from the wisdom gained in her 89+ years. I told her, "Mom, think of the aides who come to help us. They are coming to help with your care, but God is also sending *them* to *you*. You may be the one who grounds them in this life by sharing our Jesus. You might be their lifeline." She looked at me with renewed sparkle and said, "That's very true. Everyone is searching for something. He's right in front of them. They just need to believe."

- ❖ Mom just turned to me and said, "Today is National Dog Day. Do something nice for your dog."

- ❖ Mom, struggling to get out of her recliner, *(because she refuses to use the lift setting)*, "I wish you wouldn't put glue in my chair."

- ❖ I just asked Mom if she wanted a glass of cranberry juice. She looked at me, deadpan, and said, "A shot and a beer." *(Incidentally, Mom doesn't drink alcohol.)*

- ❖ Mom has a disconnect sometimes, trying to get her legs to do what her brain is telling them. She stopped, midstride with her walker, and growled, "it makes me MAD!" I said, "does it help?". She burst out laughing and said, "no".

Just Mom

In September of 2017, our area became "ground zero" for one of the most ferocious hurricanes in history, Hurricane Irma. We had never evacuated for a storm before, but we knew we needed to run this time. Mom was a big determining factor in our evacuation. We needed her to be safe with needs met. We loaded up our family and caravanned to another state. Dear friends had graciously offered up their vacation home which was large enough to house our entire clan. What might have been "the worst of times", looking back, truly became "the best of times". My mom got to have a road trip, something that she hadn't done in decades. She spent a week in a beautiful home on a lake surrounded by her family. She got to cuddle her newborn great granddaughter, my first grandchild. She referred to it daily as "a vacation". Where we saw panic and fear of the unknown *(like "would we even have a home to return to?")*, Mom simply saw time with her family in a beautiful setting, an adventure that she would talk about until her last day. Thankfully, our homes were spared. We were able to return a week later. Slowly, as life returned to normal, Mom's health began to decline.

Within a few of weeks of being home, it became obvious that we needed more help in order to meet Mom's increasing healthcare needs. We began a partnership with Hope Hospice. They were an invaluable resource and support enabling us to continue caring for Mom at home.

As I gave my son and daughter-in-law the "sleep when your newborn sleeps no matter the time of day" advice, I had no idea that my own advice would be returning to me. Mom was no longer able to get out of bed without assistance in order to use the bathroom, which meant me getting up with her a couple times during the night. *I wish I was a good napper!*

Today, Mom woke up thinking that she was in the school library (where she worked for decades as a media aide) and I'm "the nurse", but at least she recognizes Bella. Everyone should have a Bella to ground them.

- ❖ As I transfer Mom from her chair to her wheelchair and push her through the living room and into the hallway, she goes, "Weeeee!" *Hey, might as well enjoy the ride, right?*

- ❖ Mom fell last week and is still recovering with a sore back and some burning sciatic pain. Today she said, "all I can hear in my head is Johnny Cash singing that 'burning ring of fire' song."

- ❖ Mom was commenting on how tall a man was on the TV show she was watching. When she saw that he was married to a much shorter woman, she said, "Why would such a tall man want to be with such a short woman?" Then she paused and answered her own question, "Oh I know why---

because he'll always have someone who looks up to him!"

As Mom's body became weaker, she was no longer able to get out of bed. Soon, it was even difficult for her to use utensils to eat. She would struggle, determined to do it on her own, but it was exhausting for her. I encouraged her to let me help.

For the first time in my life, I fed my mom her dinner tonight. It was a bittersweet, humbling, "full-circle" moment. When she finished, she said, "Thank you for doing that. It was nice being lazy." I giggled with her and responded, "You've earned it, Mom." And she has.

Tonight, Mom and I were having our usual bedtime chat. We were talking about how many kids I have and how many kids she has, specifically daughters. Suddenly she said, "well I don't think of you as a daughter." Taken aback, slightly wounded and confused, I said, "What do you mean by that? What do you think of me as?" She responded, "You're my buddy, my best friend!" She went on to explain herself with sentiments that I will forever carry in my heart. There have been a few people who have questioned why I have chosen to be my mom's caregiver (with all that it entails) until the day she makes her final journey Home. Tonight's conversation is why. She has always been my best friend. She deserves the same and it is my honor to provide it.

❖ As I washed, dried, and curled Mom's hair today while she lay relaxing in her bed *(yes, you can have spa day even when bedridden),* she wryly quipped, "you could get a job with an undertaker!"

❖ Mom's hearing is really getting bad, worse when she's tired like tonight. We were having a serious conversation that just got more amusing as it went on. Discussing aches and pains, I said, "I'm just glad you don't hurt when you're lying in bed." Mom: "No, in the hallway." Me: "You don't go in the hallway." Mom: "No, I fell in the hallway." Me: "huh?" Mom: "What did you say?" Me: *repeats original statement. Mom: *now giggling* "I thought you said I fell in bed." Me: "No, but you're going deaf." Mom: "What?" Me: *laughing hysterically, pointing to my ears,* "Deaf! You're going DEAF." By this point we're both laughing and decide to quit while we're ahead and call it a night.

❖ Tonight, as I tuck Mom in, I say, "Ok, are you all set?" "Yes, thank you, Alex." *(Even though there are times when she may not know who I am, I ALWAYS know who she is, and that makes ALL the difference!)*

Just Mom

My husband and I had been watching Merlin on Netflix and this line really resonated with me as the tearful Merlin mourned the pending death of his dear dragon,
Merlin: "What will I do without you?" Dragon: "You will remember me."
What will I do without her?—my amazing, strong, brave Mom? What will I do without HER?
I will remember.

- ❖ Tonight, Christmas Eve, when my husband said goodnight to Mom, he said, "I'll see you in the morning. I'm off tomorrow." With her quick wit that never wanes, she quipped, "I'm always 'off'!"

- ❖ As I was donning my back-support brace before lifting Mom, she looked at me and said, "Did you earn your black belt from lifting your mother?" *(*Side note: This silly exchange was a true Christmas blessing after Mom being lost in Lewy-Body delusions for the last 36 hours!)*

Beverly Carriere Tiner

THE VALLEY OF THE SHADOW

Just Mom

God knows exactly what we need and always, always provides it. The last 24 hours have been particularly difficult with regard to my mom's Lewy-Body dementia. Lost in delusions characteristic of her disease, most of the time, she hasn't recognized me. This evening, she was a little more coherent than she's been. I told her I was making shepherd's pie tonight and she said, "Oh, *Bev* makes that! It's real good." I said, "I *am* Bev". Then she lamented about not knowing her own daughter. Then, just as quickly, she said, "another good thing she made the other day was...". Knowing she had lost me again, I said, "broccoli cheese soup?" She smiled and said "YES!". I let her rest and went to the kitchen to make dinner. Meanwhile, my husband went in her room to chat with her. He mentioned that "Bev" was making some shepherd's pie. She said, "Oh the lady that runs this place is making that tonight, too. Do you know her?" He assured her that he did.

One of the only ways I was able to survive the last couple of months, and even more so, the last couple of weeks of caring for Mom, was to separate my duties in my brain. There were times that I just had to shut off the noise emanating from my aching heart—the heart of her daughter, and just be her caregiver, nurse, advocate, and interceder. I tended to all of her needs, which eventually came to include administering morphine and other Hospice prescribed drugs.

Fast forward to after dinner. She was softly dozing. Knowing I, *her daughter*, was a bit lost to her still, I donned my *caregiver* hat, gently woke her, brushed her teeth, gave her the prescribed nighttime medications and said, "There you go! All fresh and nice for the night. I won't bother you anymore.". I thought that would be it as she was already dozing back off. Then, in her sleepy voice, she said, "You don't bother me. I love you." *Oh, how I needed that gift tonight.*

Mom is only able to eat small bites of soft things now. I asked her what sounded good to her. In her best New England accent, she quietly responded, "lobster". Thank you, Publix, for making it possible for me to spoil my mom's taste buds just a little bit more. She said it was delicious.

During Mom's brief phone conversation with my brother this morning, she told him, "Bev stopped by to feed me breakfast." After I fed her a few bites of egg, she looked at me and said, "Where are we?" I reminded her that we are at my house. I pointed out the wallpaper border that is on her bedroom wall, "Remember, Mom? You helped hang that when the girls were kids." Her response: "Yeah...that border is everywhere I go."

Some moments are so precious, you find yourself wishing for a way to hold onto them forever. If there was a way to just turn it to precious metal or sparkling gem, we would do it, yet the spirit knows even that would not capture the sweet essence of precious memories. Just such a memory was born today as my dear friend, Cathy, who was actually my mom's friend first, came to visit today. She had such a beautiful time reminiscing with Mom, even more special because Mom hasn't had this level of lucidity in days. Our friend, who also happens to be a pastor, had a time of prayer with Mom before their visit ended. Before she said amen, and quite unexpectedly, Mom added her own prayer, thanking Jesus for this time together. My heart will cherish that moment forever.

Jan 25, 2018 - This morning at 7:30, my funny, incredibly brave mom beat Lewy-Body Dementia at its own game when she stood up, strong of mind and body, and walked fearlessly into the loving arms of our Lord, Jesus Christ. Our grieving hearts will miss her beyond words during the time that we continue to tread earth's sod without her, but we do not grieve as those who have no hope.

1 Thessalonians 4:13-18 reminds us: "And now, dear brothers and sisters, we want you to know what will happen to the believers who have died so you will not grieve like people who have no hope. For since we believe that Jesus died and was raised to life again, we also believe that when Jesus returns, God will bring back with him the believers who have died. We tell you this directly from the Lord: We who are still living when the Lord returns will not meet him ahead of those who have

died. For the Lord himself will come down from heaven with a commanding shout, with the voice of the archangel, and with the trumpet call of God. First, the believers who have died will rise from their graves. Then, together with them, we who are still alive and remain on the earth will be caught up in the clouds to meet the Lord in the air. Then we will be with the Lord forever. So encourage each other with these words."

We *will* be together again. One of the last things Mom said to me was, "Don't cry. We will all be together again one day." That is the beautiful hope and promise that we cling to. The golden tie that binds our spirits to hers is not broken, only stretched a little bit longer.

I returned from running errands today to find an absolutely gorgeous floral arrangement from my church family waiting at my door. As I brought it inside and placed it in the living room where it joined a beautiful bouquet from my daughter and son-in-law and a vase of lovely flowers from my husband, I hear in my spirit a familiar cheeky voice with an ever-so-slight New England accent say: *"Boy! It looks like a funeral parlor in here!"* I can't help but smile through my tears.

Just Mom

I was in my mom's room sorting through a few things when her calendar caught my eye. My niece used to send Mom a beautiful calendar at the end of each year. Mom always looked forward to her new calendar. I used to cross the date off for her every night at bedtime in order to help her keep track of each day's passing. Today I looked at it and realized that I had stopped crossing days off *the day she crossed over.* My spirit said, "it was the day time stood still."

Holy Spirit said, "No, look at the message above the dates, on the calendar photo. That was the day her real life began."

At the top of the calendar, above a photo of beautiful, white lilies, it read:

"FROM THE END SPRINGS NEW BEGINNINGS".

Indeed.

THOUGHTS FOR THE GRIEVING AND THOSE WHO LOVE THEM

I have shared many facets of my "Mom" journey with you. I would be remiss, especially as counselor, if I did not also share something about grieving. As is true for many of us who have cared for a loved one with dementia, much of the grieving began long before my mother left this life, as, little by little, Lewy killed her. Nothing could have prepared me for life without her, though.

I told someone that my mantra is, "Give yourself permission"; "Permission to be busy. Permission to sit quietly. Permission to be alone looking at the sky, breathing in nature. Permission to stand in her room and tell her how much I miss her. Permission to wear her sweater like a hug. Permission to laugh. Permission to weep. Permission to walk the journey of healing in whatever way my soul and body need at any given moment. Permission to stretch my feelers the full length that the cord has now been stretched." As I literally felt like I was trudging through mud both physically and emotionally, I also felt peace, because I knew that God was with me in the mud. I was conscious to keep moving *through* it, not remain *stuck* in it. Grief is a slow journey and one that is as individual as a snowflake. I know many of you are also walking a path of grief today. I hope this helps you as well. We will walk together...and alone...at our own pace. And that's ok.

I have spoken to many whose mothers have died. Across the board, I hear the same sentiment: losing your mother is different than other losses. Hers was the first face you saw, the first voice you recognized. Her touch was the healing balm for all of life's ailments. She was your first love. She taught you to speak. She held your hand and taught you to walk. She walked with you throughout all of your life. Then, one fateful day, she was gone. Her spirit was called from her earthly body, the body that had perhaps been failing her for so long. She was set free, healed, whole. You were left standing still. Like a toddler unable to take another step for fear of falling, you reached for your mother's hand, only to find that she was not there. Suddenly you couldn't move.

This is what it feels like when your mother dies. We all experience loss in this life and if you haven't yet, sadly, you will. It is part of the journey. We all edge our way Home. Some get there before others. It is the natural order of things. I thought, having already witnessed the passing of my father and others whom I loved, that my mother's passing and the following time of grieving would be pretty much the same. I was wrong. It was not the same at all. Many who have walked closely with their moms and later become their caregivers have agreed. Our psyches are so linked with our mothers that we feel as though a spiritual amputation has taken place.

When our mothers cross over, part of us goes with them. It is more than a "normal grieving", if there even is such a thing. It is a gut-punch to our entire being. It is a shifting of the sand beneath our feet. It is an untethering. It hurts to our core, but it is so much more than that. We are left, like that toddler, having to figure out how to take that next step without her hand there to guide us, to catch us should we stumble.

We are left to make a choice. We can stand still or barrel forward. I advise the standing still for a bit. Even sit down right in that spot if need be. It's impossible to move forward when you can't catch your breath. The breathing in and breathing out was once shared with this amazing person. Now it's just you. So, sit and practice for a while. Cry and breathe for as long as it takes. Let me warn you: You will *not*, one day, pop up and start running. You will be more like a baby deer with shaky newborn legs. You will, one day, attempt to stand and you will fall right back down. And that's okay. Sit a while longer.

At some point, you will make another attempt to stand and your legs won't feel so shaky. You might even take a couple of steps. You will find it exhausting. Did you know that grief makes you tired? It also hurts. You may notice that you have more aches and pains than normal.

That's because your entire being just got hit by a truck. Take care of your physical self as well as your emotional and spiritual self. It's more important now than ever that you treat yourself like you would your best friend. Be patient with *you*.

That brings me to my next thought. Perhaps a couple of weeks have passed since your mom went Home. You actually feel worse. What? Yes, you do. That's because you've been so busy handling the affairs that come with one's passing, that your heart hasn't even had time to catch up. Maybe it's been a month, or two. You're still randomly bursting into tears. You still can't bear to clean out her closet. Six months have passed. You still can't listen to her favorite song, still bury your nose in her pillow when no one is looking--the pillow that you can't throw away. Perhaps it's been a year. You've marked every holiday as the first one without her. Two years…four…ten, *even more*. We never stop missing our mothers. There is no perfect timetable for grief. Each journey is unique. There is no right way to do it.

We make a mistake asking, "when will life get back to normal?". The answer is, "never". If we have surgery on part of our body, we are left with a scar. We learn to live with that scar. We know that our bodies will never be as they were pre-surgery. It is the same with this level of loss. When our moms die, we are forever changed. That doesn't mean that life will not be good--even great again.

It doesn't mean that we won't be happy. It means that life will be different. It will not be as it once was. Stop expecting that to happen. In time, we will find our new footing. Jesus promises us abundant life. He doesn't say "mediocre" life. (John 10:10) Do not expect things to be as they once were. Look forward to what He has in store for you now. *Different, yet abundant.*

Here's the thing: our moms are the life-givers, the ones who chose to birth us, nurture us, love us. They are likely the first ones who taught us what unconditional love meant. When they leave their earthly bodies behind, the golden cord that has bound us is stretched to the point that, to our finite minds, it feels as though it's been severed. It is like the hose that once provided our oxygen supply from the tank next to our bodies has now been stretched to the house next door. We struggle to breathe until we learn a new way. Dear one, that cord that binds us to our mothers is not snipped. It is stretched. So, breathe a little more slowly until you get the hang of it.

Find your own way to move forward and in your own time. Each day try to take a baby step. Change your routine a bit. Change will help to rewire your brain. If you need a day off in between, that's okay, too. Spend time with Jesus. Really. I'm not being cliché here. You will find a deep reserve of strength that He is holding for just this time. It is yours and you need it. You access it through Him. That is precisely why He said, "Come to

Me all you who are heavy laden." (Matthew 11:28) Come to Him. Let Him hold you. He will teach you, ever so gently, how to take those steps without her.

And finally, a quick word to those who wish to comfort grieving friends or family members; please choose your words carefully. A gentle hug and affectionate word is enough. A long recounting of your own experience is not generally comforting. To the grieving heart, this is akin to being held hostage. Don't do it (unless asked). Saying that you know just how they feel is also not helpful--because, no matter how similar your own experience may be, you, in fact, do *not* know how they feel. This is *their* grief journey. Respect it. Be a little gentler, a little more kind. Keep an eye on your loved one. Don't expect them to jump right back into life. They are likely more fragile than they are letting on. Pray for them often. Send a text, a card, make a short call. They are in a battle like no other. They need you, not so much your sympathy--just *you*. They are, after all, just learning how to walk again *and it's really, really hard.*

www.ingramcontent.com/pod-product-compliance
Lightning Source LLC
Chambersburg PA
CBHW072231170526
45158CB00002BA/854